OMAHA PUBLIC LIBRARY

DEC   2014

The Sinusitis And Headaches Solution

Steps To Relieve Sinus, Common Cold And Headaches

D1310821

Rossie C Pattison

Copyright Notice

Copyright © 2014 Rossie C Pattison. All Rights Reserved.

All rights reserved. No part of this publication may be reproduced, distributed, or transmitted in any form or by any means, including photocopying, recording, or other electronic or mechanical methods, without the prior written permission of the publisher, except in the case of brief quotations embodied in critical reviews and certain other non-commercial uses permitted by copyright law.

This book is a general educational health-related information product. As an express condition to reading this book, you understand and agree to the following terms. The books content is not a substitute for direct, personal, professional medical care and diagnosis.

Please see your doctor or health care provider if you are unsure of eating any of the foods in this book or participating in any of the activities as everyone has different health care needs and concerns.

The Author and/ or Publisher of this book is not responsible in any manner whatsoever for any consequential damages that result from the use of, or the inability to use this book.

First Printing, 2014

ISBN-13: 978-1497504806

CONTENTS

INTRODUCTION

Sinusitis, Headaches And Deafness

These facts about sinusitis, deafness, and headaches may come as news to you

THE head, "home of the brain," can be afflicted with troubles ranging all the way from the unpleasantness of a burning tongue to the agony of migraine headache. Between the two pain extremes are the ear disorders that may bring on loss of hearing, and the sinus infections that may be anything from uncomfortable to injurious to the general health because of hidden germ pockets.

Although the disorders and maladies of the head rarely prove fatal in themselves, they can "kill" the joy of living for their victims.

Ache for ache, head troubles can cause more chronic misery than almost any other part of the body. Yet no group of ailments is more promisingly preventable, even curable, through common sense and good nutrition than most of these "miseries" of the head.

Few of them fail to show at least some improvement under a regimen of proper diet, common sense and nutritional therapy.

The head is the "port of entry" for infections

The virus of the common cold is believed to sneak into the bloodstream via a weak spot in the mucous membrane lining of the nose or throat. His relative the pneumococcus instigator of pneumonia finds its way to the base of operations (the lungs) down the tender, membrane-lined upper respiratory tract.

And the other viruses and bacteria, whose number is legion, also find the nose, mouth and throat their most convenient port of entry. These sites are moist and warm, a spot where a hard-working virus or germ can be sure of a welcome, especially if the foolish mortal to whom these parts belong has allowed his resistance to fall way below normal because of undue fatigue, overindulgence in food or alcohol, chilling, emotional upsets or excess accumulations of stagnant mucus.

However, it is not always the germs and viruses that send patients scurrying to the doctor for treatment.

The offices of nose and throat specialists are filled with patients who show no physical signs to account for their head disorders. Here again the mind proves its power to stir up trouble with the physical organs.

A famous head specialist stated recently that, while some of the patients who visit their doctor for relief of head symptoms are victims of genuine physical disorders, the general run of sufferers were those whose thinking is faulty and whose emotions prevent personal adjustment to changing circumstances.

CHAPTER 1 – The Human Ear

The hearing apparatus the human ear is one of the most wonderful precision instruments ever devised. It is divided into the outer, the middle and the inner ear. The outer ear is the trumpet-like appendage set on either side of the head to collect and transmit to the inner ear the sound vibrations received from the air.

The middle ear amplifies these vibrations into what are called "lymph" waves. And the inner ear transforms the lymph vibrations into a nervous impulse which allows the brain to translate into thought sensations the vibrations which the ear has "heard."

Where the auditory canal, leading inward from the outer ear, meets the middle ear is stretched the eardrum. Inflammations that affect the middle ear (a space as large as a pea) usually result from a catarrhal condition caused by colds and grippe, or by infectious diseases such as measles.

Earache is caused when the pus from this infection of the middle ear backs up behind the eardrum and causes pressure on the delicate ear nerves. The eardrum is a strong membrane, with fibers so elastic that it can expand and contract under the impact of air pressure.

However, unusually strong sound vibrations, such as claps of thunder or heavy explosions may bring so much pressure to bear on this membrane that it will rupture.

If a loud noise can be anticipated, opening the mouth wide will equalize the pressure on both sides of the eardrum, thereby preventing rupture of the auricular membrane.

Besides the two tiny organs of equilibrium that enable us to maintain a sense of upright body position, the inner ear also contains the cochlea, the specific hearing instrument which is constructed with "strings" and "sounding board" miraculously similar to a piano.

Within this cochlea are suspended auditory cells; and each of these auditory cells is surrounded by a network of nerve endings leading to nerve "cables" that enter the center channels of the cochlea direct from the brain.

To provide nourishment for these auditory cells, the walls of the cochlea are laced with arteries. Ordinarily, a deaf ear is one whose nerve "cables" are short-circuited, or whose auditory cells are starving for nourishment.

In the three parts of the human hearing apparatus outer, middle and inner ear all the canals, chambers and recesses, as well as the Eustachian tube leading into the nose and throat from the middle ear, are lined with mucous membranes.

Improper diet can cause these mucous membranes in the delicate hearing apparatus to swell and congest.

And when this marvelous instrument is distorted, swollen and congested with stagnant blood, it can no more send perfect sound impressions to the brain than a radio with defective tubes can receive non-distorted broadcast waves. A good sense of hearing depends upon healthy auditory cells and nerves.

Where the hearing instrument has been damaged by injury or

infection, deafness is usually difficult to overcome. However, when the loss of hearing is purely functional, much can be done by the victim to relieve his condition.

CHAPTER 2 - Deafness

Deafness is a very stealthy disease; often it sneaks upon its victim so gradually that it is not noticed until a good part of the hearing is gone. How deaf is "deafness"? If the hearing is even so little as 5 percent below normal, deafness has set in and the wise person will take immediate steps to halt progression of the disease, even though the lost 5 percent of hearing may, or may not, be restorable.

It is a tragic error to think that the ability to hear "some sounds" does not mean that the ear is becoming deaf; it is foolhardy to wait until all hearing is gone before attempting to do something about deaf-ness.

About 90 percent of all deafness results from nasal catarrh. Head specialists say that deafness would be a rare ailment if all nasal and sinus troubles were treated early enough before they involved the delicate ear mechanisms.

As this type of deafness responds slowly, if ever, to therapy of any type, it is wise to start clearing up all nasal and sinus disorders before infections are able to invade the organs of the inner ear.

However, for certain types of deafness that are related to deficient nerve functioning, nutritional therapy offers the brightest hope of prevention and relief that has yet been discovered. Dormant nerve "cables" in the cochlea can be revived by giving the patient a combination of selected vitamins and amino acids in pure, concentrated form. This treatment, developed by Drs.

Hans Hirschfeld, Max Jacobson and Augusta Jellinek of New York, was tried on 78 deaf persons. One of them, a thirty seven year old man who had shown a progressive loss of hearing for 15 years, had been discharged from the Army because of his deafness.

Both ears were affected; his hearing loss was 37 percent for ordinary speech and 63 percent for general sounds. After only six treatments with this combination of pure vitamins and amino acids, the man's hearing loss was reduced to 26 percent for speech and 48 percent for general sounds!

In a fifteen year boy whose loss of hearing had progressed to 54 percent, the deafness was decreased to only 1.2 percent. Some of the patients showed hearing gains of 40 percent to 50 percent, with much more for pure tones. Especially did this vitamin and amino acid therapy restore the ability to hear high tones, usually the first sounds to disappear when deafness sets in.

The vitamins contained in the capsules given in these experiments were A, C and B-complex; while the amino acids were glutamic acid, histidine and methionine. Urea was also added to the dose. Each day three of these capsules were given by mouth.

The doctors who devised this vitamin-amino acid treatment for deafness believe that these food elements act as a highly nourishing nerve food and accelerator of nerve growth.

In this report, issued by the American Medical Association, they state: "The special significance of the new compound lies in its direct influence on the stimulation and the restitution of the function of the auditory nerve itself."

CHAPTER 3 - Nutritional Treatment

The only thing new about this nutritional treatment for deafness is the amino acids, since Dr. Grant Selfridge of San Francisco has been using large amounts of vitamin B-complex for several years to check deafness and restore hearing in cases of partial deafness.

The addition of the amino acids to this already promising treatment offers greater hope than ever for certain types of deafness, since there seems to be a powerful co-operation between these vitamins and these amino acids that confers a marked beneficial effect on starved auditory nerve cells.

It would also seem logical that this same treatment of vitamins and amino acids could accomplish the same beneficial results for most victims of deafness brought on by nervous and emotional disturbances, inasmuch as these food elements nourish not only the auditory nerve, but the entire nerve structure throughout the body as well.

Perhaps it may be that serious lack of these very food elements in the first place brought on the unstable nervous or mental condition that ended by affecting the delicate ear mechanism.

You will note that one of the amino acids contained in this new nutritional treatment for deafness is glutamic acid, the food element we met earlier in this book when it was increasing the brain power in dramatic experiments undertaken with subnormal children, and raising normal intelligence to that of the "near genius" level in other children.

For this reason, I am inclined to believe that this vitamin-amino acid treatment devised by the New York doctors will also work in cases of deafness where there is a definite mental or emotional angle.

Adding these vitamins and amino acids to diets marked by their deficiency might very possibly reverse the degenerative nerve process, thereby restoring the nervous system, including the auditory nerves, to health.

The ear, like many other parts of the body, seldom, if ever, gets any exercise. That is why blood circulation within the ear is likely to be poor. To a large extent this can be overcome by performing a simple little exercise once a day.

Take the lobe of the ear between the thumb and forefinger and pull down very gently 10 times, releasing the lobe after each little tug. Besides stimulating the flow of blood to the ear, this gentle motion tends also to loosen any accumulations of hardening wax that often cause the hearing to become defective.

To those wearers of false teeth and partial plates, I want to impart a word of warning: About six million deaf or hard of hearing persons in the United States can thank poorly fitted dentures for the damage to their inner ear.

Dr. Goodfriend of the University of Pennsylvania reported in the Archives of Otolaryngology that a faulty bite caused by ill-fitting false teeth or plates causes some kinds of deafness. Patients who had complained of ear troubles were completely relieved after he had straightened their teeth.

Further, he noticed that various types of headaches which had been diagnosed as "tic douloureux" or "tumors of the brain" seemed to clear up completely after the faulty dentures were corrected to allow a meeting of the upper and lower teeth in a proper bite.

Dr. Goodfriend cited the case history of a fifty eight year old watchman in Philadelphia who complained to his doctors about acute dizziness, nausea and increasing deafness.

At two different hospitals the watchman's ailment was diagnosed as arising from two vastly different causes: one specialist suggested a gall bladder operation, while the other specialist maintained that the trouble was caused by a brain tumor.

Finally, a dentist proposed that the man be given a good set of false teeth before anything as drastic as surgery was undertaken.

Thanks to the common sense of that dentist and his simple diagnosis, the watchman's symptoms disappeared. His deafness cleared up and, of course, he did not have to submit to any experimental operations.

When the teeth do not meet properly in a "good bite," the dentists call it malocclusion. A faulty bite raises the jaw, which in turn tips the head of the jawbone so that, instead of sliding comfortably into its normal pocket under the ear, the tilted jawbone presses on the outer ear passage, the Eustachian tube, as well as on the muscles, nerves, blood vessels and other extremely delicate apparatus of the inner ear.

After a while, this faulty bite will cause the mechanism of the ear to deteriorate, bringing on symptoms of dizziness, ringing in the ears and progressively worse deafness. So please, for the sake of your hearing, seek the services of the best dental surgeon available when false teeth or partial plates are absolutely necessary.

As revealed in a national women's magazine recently, there are too many "bootleg dentists" in the United States today who pass off an eagerness for quick profit as skilled crafts manship.

Poorly or indifferently trained dental mechanics by the hundreds are turning out dentures which are nothing short of criminal, and for which the patient is asked to pay an exorbitant price. (In all fairness to American dental schools, let it be said that a great majority of these "bootleg" dental mechanics are foreign trained men lately arrived in this country.)

Many ear infections, as well as cases of so-called "pocket handkerchief deafness," could be avoided if the nose were properly blown. Clamping both nostrils tightly shut between the handkerchief, then causing a forceful blast through the closed nostrils reacts against the eardrums, and may even cause a rupture of this membrane.

Or, continual blowing in this manner many stretches the eardrum membrane so that it can no longer be tensed enough to receive fine vibrations of air—hence the hearing is dulled.

Further, this foolish way of blowing the nose also forces bacteria and foreign matter up the Eustachian tube from the middle throat into the inner ear. In fact, many earaches start from infections that travel via this route from the throat upward into the ears.

If you must blow your nose, press the handkerchief lightly against only one nostril at a time, making sure to open the mouth wide while doing so. This helps equalize the pressure on both sides of the eardrum.

But a recent bulletin issued by the Army Medical Department goes a step further and advises that if you have a common cold, don't blow your nose, be a sniffer!

Forceful inhalation or sniffing is the only safe way to clear the nose, according to this authority. "This habit (blowing with nostrils closed) must be broken," declares the bulletin, "because blowing creates positive pressure in the upper respiratory passages.

There is always a certain amount of secretion about the small openings of the nasal sinuses which is forced back into the sinuses by blowing."

Dizziness and deafness appearing together must be suspected of being symptoms of an ear disturbance known as Meniere's disease. Other symptoms that often accompany this disorder of the inner ear are head noises and vomiting.

The site of the disturbance is in the extremely delicate organs of balance located in the inner ear; these are the tiny organs that enable us to keep our equilibrium.

In other words, without these sensitive organs in each ear, we would walk head down toward the ground, and never have any knowledge of what position the body was in at a particular moment.

In severe cases of Meniere's disease, the victim may suddenly be seized with such extreme dizziness that he staggers and falls to the ground like one under the influence of alcohol.

Then again, the dizziness may be noticed only when turning the head, or when rolling over in bed. Sometimes the victim suffers two or three attacks, and then the symptoms disappear, never to return. Others, however, are not so lucky, and the annoying symptoms continue for months, even years.

The discomfort of Meniere's disease results when the small semi-circular canals of the inner ear become congested and swell, thus throwing the organs of balance out of line. Blame for this swelling of the auricular canals in the inner ear is placed on several things.

The tiny blood vessels supplying the inner ear may become constricted, one cause of this constriction being continued exposure to chills or drafts that tend to contract the neck muscles, thereby congesting the blood vessels and diminishing the flow of blood to the ears.

An allergic reaction to some food or external substance in the air may also cause this congestion. A nest of infection in the nose, throat, sinuses, tonsils or teeth may allow germs to invade the inner ear.

Plenty of rest and a low starch diet are indicated in any kind of ear disturbance, and especially in Meniere's disease. Niacin and thiamin (both members of the vitamin B-complex group) have been used successfully to relieve the unpleasant symptoms of this ear disorder. Swelling of the ear canals is often reduced when the victim is put on a salt-free diet.

In fact, table salt may cause the mucous membranes of the upper respiratory tract to retain water. After a month or so of either a salt-free diet, or one low in sodium chloride, marked improvement has also been noted in various types of deafness, as well as in sinusitis and chronic colds.

CHAPTER 4 - Table Salt

Healthy Nasal and Head Passages

Table salt often interferes with the body's use of calcium. When it is eliminated from the diet, calcium metabolism is frequently restored to normal, thus accounting for the relief conferred by salt-free diets in these types of head disorders.

The nose is a filter, lined with thousands of tiny nostril hairs, set in a line of mucous membrane. All the recesses and chambers of the nose, as well as those leading back into the skull, called sinuses, are lined with a covering of mucous membrane so that blood "on the instant" can be supplied when the nose is called upon to warm air before it enters the lungs.

In winter, or when entering a cold room, more blood is pumped to the nose passages, causing the mucous membrane linings to swell, thus narrowing the space through which the chilled air must pass.
This accounts for the fact that the nose seems to become

unaccountably congested on a warm day when remaining for any length of time in an air-conditioned building.

The change from warm to cool is so sudden that emergency supplies of blood are rushed to the nasal membranes in order that the overly chilled air cannot reach the lungs before it is warmed. And this sudden rush of blood to the mucous membrane causes nasal congestion.

Obviously, healthy nasal and head passages (sinuses) depend upon healthy mucous membranes. These membranes, when in good condition, secrete natural substances that are a powerful germicide against bacteria and viruses that enter the nasal passages via the air.

As stated earlier in this chapter, these nasal passages are a "port of entry" for infectious organisms. But wherever nature has provided a body opening, she has also equipped that opening with a mucous membrane lining so that it may secrete this natural germicidal substance to protect the body from bacterial invaders.

The eye sockets and the eyelids, for instance, are lined with mucous membranes, and the eye secretion (tears) is another germicide.

If these mucous membranes that line the various body openings are properly nourished (and vitamin A seems to be one of the specific food elements that contributes toward a healthy mucous membrane), and if they are kept free from accumulations of excess mucus that prevent free flow of the germ-killing secretions, then the body opening is well fortified against bacteria and virus invaders.

But a poorly nourished mucus-coated nasal passage is a weak opening, in poor condition to resist the constant onslaught of the millions of germ invaders inhaled with every breath. This accounts for the wave of colds, grippe and influenza that can be depended upon to break out around the holiday season every year.

Too many rich viands, not enough high-vitamin foods and insufficient rest, coupled with inhaling smoke-polluted air all contribute toward weakening the membranous linings of the nasal and throat passages.

And when these passages drop so far below normal strength that a weak spot occurs, the cold virus and the flu and pneumonia germs pour into the bloodstream by the millions through this gap in the mucous membrane wall.

In other words, your resistance to chronic colds, sore throat, and other infections of the upper respiratory tract and lungs is no stronger than the mucous membranes that line your nose and throat.

One common outgrowth of the chronic cold is "sinus trouble." Chronic catarrh of the nasal passages allows infection to creep back into the winding sinuses where its eradication is usually a long, slow, painful process.

Anyone who has ever experienced the heavy pressure headaches that accompany sinusitis knows that the best remedy for sinus infection is prevention. Usually, if the catarrhal condition of the nasal passages can be cleared up early enough, the symptoms of sinus infection will also disappear.

But if allowed to run on, sinus infections, with their constant discharge of poisonous matter into the digestive tract, may lead to such diseases as arthritis, gall bladder infection or pneumonia.

Excess table salt in the diet aggravates chronic nasal catarrh; frequently, when the use of salt is cut to an absolute minimum, the pains of sinusitis are relieved and the infection clears up.

Another word of advice to sinus sufferers as well as to all victims of "head troubles" is to omit heavy starches and white sugars from the diet. For sweetening, honey is recommended as a more than satisfactory substitute, since the chemical composition of honey makes it a good remedy in itself for nasal and sinus congestions.

Plenty of sleep, rest and fresh air are necessary in the treatment of any bodily disorder, and sinus infection is no exception. Keeping the body clean internally is also essential to clearing up all infections.

If waste matter from both the infected area and from the intestines is not eliminated from the body according to a normal schedule, these noxious substances take up residence in the bloodstream and further aggravate any existing catarrhal or allergic disorder. Proper elimination can be aided in victims of sinusitis by following a Purifying Diet.

CHAPTER 5 - Diet

Fruit juices, distilled or mineral water, and an herb tea such as that brewed from fenugreek, help cleanse the system of excess mucus or other impurities. Sinus infection and the type of eye disorders brought on by a diet poor in vitamin A seem to go hand in hand.

The explanation for this is that any diet so low in vitamin A that it affects the eyes will also starve the mucous membranes of the throat and nasal passages, predisposing the victim toward chronic colds; and, after a more or less extended bout with the cold virus, the way is paved for infection of the sinuses.

Many sinus patients find this "cocktail" a good way to get extra vitamins into the diet, in addition to those obtained in the meals, and in concentrated form.

Once a week, into a glass two-thirds full of tomato juice, grate about a tablespoonful of horseradish root (purchased fresh in the market, not the kind already grated and bottled in vinegar).

Wrap the balance of the root in waxed paper and put away in a cool place to be used in succeeding weeks. This tomato juice-horseradish cocktail is used by many of those sinusitis victims who follow my health regimen and their reports are enthusiastic about this tonic as an addition to a sane dietary program.

Even many of the physicians specializing in disorders of the head now concede that operations for sinusitis can do no good, and may cause irreparable damage.

The best treatment for sinus disorders, in their opinion, is to raise the general bodily resistance to a high level by obtaining plenty of rest, drinking ample fruit and vegetable juices, and following a high vitamin diet supplemented with large doses of vitamin A in concentrated form and in this they confirm what I have been teaching for years!

One other organ of the head is likely to protest when nutrition of the entire body falls below normal, and that is the tongue. Anyone who has ever experienced a sore, swollen, burning tongue knows the misery this upset can bring. Because the tongue is a good indicator (otherwise doctors would not be so interested in seeing it), any change in its appearance usually means something is wrong elsewhere in the body.

Whenever the tongue begins to burn, many persons know they are "in for" their periodic spell of anemia, and they begin taking iron and liver concentrate.

A tender, slick, swollen, beefy-red tongue may also indicate a need for the niacin and riboflavin contained in vitamin B-complex. But sometimes a sore, burning tongue is the result of unbalanced diets undertaken either as a fad, or as a relief for an intestinal disturbance. Or the tongue may be irritated by broken, irregular teeth, or ill-fitting dentures.

It has also been noted that teeth fillings of two different metals can create an electrical current that affects the tongue. Some persons have found their tongues becoming red and sore after being fitted with plastic dentures.

Moreover, a burning tongue may be caused by some nervous disorder, since many persons complain of this symptom only during periods of anxiety or aggravated unrest. This disorder has been known to show up in women during the menopause and in men during their climacteric.

Another cause for a sore, swollen tongue can be traced to a disturbance of the salivary glands. Either the saliva is insufficient, or it becomes thickened and accumulates in strings stretching from the soft palate to the tongue.

When trouble with the tongue arises from the salivary glands, liberal amounts of fluids, particularly the cleansing, stimulating teas made from mild herbs, are remarkably beneficial.

The tongue also brings attention to itself by being the seat of the taste glands. Anyone who has ever been deprived of the innumerable joys that a good sense of taste entails knows how important to pleasurable living it is to keep the taste buds in good condition.

During a severe head cold, for example, the sense of taste and smell also may be lost. This is because heavy secretions from the membranes of the nose and mouth have buried the taste buds (as well as the nerves of smell in the nose) under a blanket of excess mucus.

And it is this unwanted coating of mucus and other impurities that cuts off the taste buds in the tongue from intimate contact with the food taken into the mouth. Anyone suffering from chronic catarrh of the nasal or sinus passages almost always experiences a loss or dulling of his senses of taste and smell.

Keeping the mouth cleansed frequently with a mild mouthwash that will dissolve mucus will help restore the sense of taste. However, a strong mouthwash is to be avoided, especially one containing a high percentage of alcohol.

The safest, mildest mucus-solvent for the mouth, nose and throat that I have found is one made from my favorite herb, fenugreek. The taste is pleasant, and the action is mild. In fact, in our home we find a tea brewed from fenugreek is one of our best standbys against ordinary head disorders such as the common cold and sore throat.

Space will not permit dwelling at length on another type of head disturbance, migraine. However, I do want to mention that research has found many cases of this torturing type of headache are caused by emotional disturbances.

Migraine and mental upsets seem to go together, since most migraine sufferers exhibit rather tense personalities. Therefore, the one way to ward off the disabling attacks of migraine is to impress upon the victim the need to remove or to avoid all situations that cause emotional tension.

Since undue emotional sensitivity is usually a feature of a nerve disorder, extraordinary results have been obtained by treating migraine with thiamin and niacin, of the vitamin B-complex group.

A certain tendency toward allergy also seems to accompany susceptibility to migraine. In one patient, it was noted that a skin rash broke out on her arms and neck every time she suffered an attack of migraine.

Finally, through observation and careful elimination of certain food items from the diet, this patient discovered that one piece of chocolate candy or a portion of Roquefort cheese was enough to bring on the skin rash and the migraine.

After eliminating these two items (of which she was inordinately fond) from the diet, she suffered no further attacks of migraine. Wisely, this patient fortified herself as a further precaution by including concentrated vitamin B-complex and amino acids in her daily diet.

Dr. Williams of the Mayo Clinic has found that one kind of headache, which formerly was considered a "sinus" headache, is actually caused by allergic reactions of certain head muscles. He calls this type of head disorder "myalgia," meaning muscle headache.

The treatment he has found most effective for this malady consists of large doses of the vitamin niacin, contained in B-complex. Perhaps no other part of the body responds so well to the sensible treatment of balanced diet, plenty of rest, good personal hygiene and dietary supplements as does the head with its "cranky" mechanisms of hearing, smelling, tasting and seeing. But to neglect and mistreat this home of the brain is to head for trouble.

CHAPTER 6

Jucing Recipes For Sinus, Common Cold And Headaches

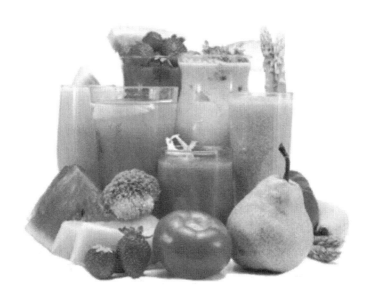

Juicing for Health

Juicing boosts the entire body, it's delicious, a great way to give your taste buds a treat. Juicing is by far one of the quickest, most delicious and best ways to get all the daily vitamins and mineral your body needs.

A recent research shows that the healthiest foods for the body are those that are easily digested. Then this concept only stands to the reason that juicing is the most effective and the best way to obtain a healthy and balanced nutritional intake daily.

When fruits and vegetables are used in making juice, the vitamins and minerals found in them are preserved, and because there's little digestion required for all these nutrients, the effects are felt instantly throughout the body.

After drinking a glass of fresh and delicious juice your energy will increase, because the fruits and vegetables are all natural the body will quickly absorbed it.

In addition, your body will have the ability to get a concentrated amount of enzymes from the fruits and vegetables when used for juicing. The enzymes are quickly taken into the body and helps in the conversion of foods into energy and body tissue.

The more enzymes the body takes in, the more efficient your digestion is likely to be and therefore the more efficient your metabolic rate will be too.

This contributes to an enhanced digestive system, less fat buildup and more effective wastes removal process. Also consuming a fresh glass of fruits and vegetables consistently will guarantee that your body gets the correct amount of phyto-chemicals, which are essential components in the body's ability in combating illness and disorders.

With all the great things juicing has to offer, it should be part of your day-to-day lifestyle. Besides from the benefits of juicing, there are other things to know, such as, how to store your juice after juicing. Always remember that it's advisable to drink juice immediately because all the nutrients and enzymes are in their freshest and purest form.

Nutmeg Elixir

Ingredients:

4 apples
2 parsnips
3 teaspoons of nutmeg

Direction:

Wash all the ingredients

Cut and core the apples. Chop up the parsnips and add all the ingredients as well as the nutmeg in the juicer. Blend for one minute.

Rhubarb Juice

Health Benefits:

Rhubarb is effective in promoting internal health. In addition, rhubarb contains lots of nutritional elements such as vitamin K, vitamin C, calcium potassium, magnesium and thiamin. Rhubarb is high in vitamin C and dietary fiber.

Ingredients:

4 large apples
7 large carrots
1 lb of cranberries
1 stalk of rhubarb

Direction:

Wash all the ingredients

Trim the ends off of the rhubarb and remove any leaves, cut and core the apples. Begin adding the ingredients to the juicer one at a time. Add ice cubes if desired and drink immediately.

Watercress Cleanse

Health Benefits:

Watercress flushes out impurities from the body; it is a seasonal vegetable that is full of antioxidants, protein, as well as vitamin b5. Stimulating salivary, gastric secretions and the regulation of the intestines tract. Packed with important nutrients watercress has folic, protein, copper, riboflavin, manganese, potassium, thiamin, vitamin A, vitamin C, vitamin E, and vitamin b 6 in it.

Ingredients:

2 watercress stalks
1 stalk of broccoli
3 cups of spinach
3 oranges

Direction:

Wash all the ingredients

Cut up the broccoli florets and place them inside the juicer then cut up the spinach and watercress into small pieces to fit in the juicer. Next peel and cut the oranges into small sections. Place the ingredients in one at a time.

Lime Detox

Ingredients:

8 tablespoons of honey
4 white grapes
1 liter water
1 lime

Direction:

Wash all the ingredients

Peel and cut the lime into 4 small pieces. Place all the ingredients into the juicer and mix until the mixture is smooth. Add ice cubes if needed.

Ginger Root Delight

Health Benefits:

A great cure for nausea, sinus and stomach upset, ginger is good for inducing blood circulation throughout the body.

Ingredients:

2 oranges
1 pineapple
ginger root   (a small piece)

Direction:

Wash all the ingredients

Remove the crown and base from pineapple and carefully cut the rind off the pineapple. Next, chop the pineapple into chunky pieces and set aside. Peel the skin from the oranges and slice into small sections to fit into the juicer. Now cut up the ginger root into smaller pieces and place all the ingredients into the juicer. Begin juicing. Drink immediately.

Kale Morning Glory

Ingredients:

2 cups of kale
1 grapefruit
2 green apples
1 cup of blueberries
4 stalks of celery

Direction:

Wash all the ingredients

Cut and core the apples, kale and celery. Peel the grapefruit and cut in small pieces to fit easily into the juicer. Process all the ingredients in the juicer.

Cabbage Juice

Ingredients:

1/ 2 of cabbage
5 almonds
3 oranges

Direction:

Wash all the ingredients

Slice the cabbage into 4 quarters, peel and cut the orange into small pieces to easily fit into the juicer. Then add the almonds and all the other ingredients to the juicer. Mix until the mixture is smooth.

Blueberry And Cantaloupe Juice

Ingredients:

1/ 2 cantaloupe
1 cup of blueberries
3 apples

Direction:

Wash all the ingredients

Peel the apple and remove the core and then cut the netted skin off of the cantaloupe. Place all the ingredients into the juicer. Add ice cubes if desired and drink immediately.

Parsnip Juice

Ingredients:

1 teaspoon of nutmeg
2 Parsnips
4 Apples

Direction:

Wash all the ingredients

Cut the apples, parsnips and the nutmeg. Add all the ingredients inside the juicer. Blend until smooth and drink immediately.

Pineapple Flush

Ingredients:

1/ 2 of pineapple
2 bananas
3 oranges

Direction:

Wash all the ingredients

Cut off the top and bottom of the pineapple. Remove the rind and cut in halves. Peel and slice the banana and orange in small chunks. Add all the ingredients into the juicer. Add ice cubes and drink immediately.

Zucchini Juice

Ingredients:

1 tbsp. of honey
1 cup of zucchini
1 cup butternut squash

Direction:

Wash all the ingredients

Remove the skin from the zucchini and butternut squash and chop into small chunks. Begin to put all the ingredients into the juicer one at a time. Blend until smooth and drink immediately.

Vegetable Blues

Ingredients:

6 carrots
12 brussels sprouts
1/ 2 lemon
6 Jerusalem artichokes
3 cups of green beans

Direction:

Wash all the ingredients

Cut off the artichoke's stem, then chop up the artichokes, green beans and carrots. Now pull off the dry leaves and put into the juicer. Peel the lemon and cut into half. Now start adding all of the ingredients to the juicer. Blend until smooth. Drink immediately.

Garlic Blues

Ingredients:

2 beets
1 clove of garlic
6 carrots
6 cups of watercress
2 red onions

Direction:

Wash all the ingredients

Remove the skin from the onions, beets and garlic and cut into chunks. Chop up the watercress. Now place all of the ingredients into the juicer. Serve in a tall glass and drink immediately.

34240694R00028

Made in the USA
Charleston, SC
03 October 2014